YOUR KNOWLEDGE HAS VALUE

- We will publish your bachelor's and
  master's thesis, essays and papers

- Your own eBook and book -
  sold worldwide in all relevant shops

- Earn money with each sale

Upload your text at www.GRIN.com
and publish for free

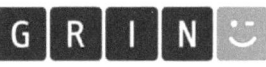

Bibliographic information published by the German National Library:

The German National Library lists this publication in the National Bibliography; detailed bibliographic data are available on the Internet at http://dnb.dnb.de .

Imprint:

Copyright © 2017 GRIN Verlag, Open Publishing GmbH
Print and binding: Books on Demand GmbH, Norderstedt Germany
ISBN: 9783668441231

This book at GRIN:

http://www.grin.com/en/e-book/358104/basic-cardiovascular-physiology

MJ Adeniyi

Basic Cardiovascular Physiology

A presentation

GRIN Publishing

GRIN - Your knowledge has value

Since its foundation in 1998, GRIN has specialized in publishing academic texts by students, college teachers and other academics as e-book and printed book. The website www.grin.com is an ideal platform for presenting term papers, final papers, scientific essays, dissertations and specialist books.

LECTURE NOTE
ON
BASIC CARDIOVASULAR PHYSIOLOGY
BY
MJ ADENIYI, MSC
DEPARTMENT OF PHYSIOLOGY
UNIVERSITY OF BENIN, BENIN-CITY
NIGERIA

INTRODUCTION

The cardiovascular system consists majorly of tubular structures called blood vessels and a muscular organ called the heart.

BLOOD VESSELS

- Histologically, blood vessels are made up of three layers; the **tunica adventitia** (outer layer), the **tunica media** (middle layer) and the **tunica intima** (the innermost layer).

- The tunica adventitia is composed of protein fibers such as elastin and collagen. These afford flexibility, shape and strength to the vessels.

- The tunica media is made up of multi-unit smooth muscle. Vagal and sympathetic stimulations of this layer bring about relaxation and constriction.

Continuation
- The tunica intima is in contact with vascular fluid and contains a single layer of endothelial cells. Endothelial cells play important role in the control of vascular permeability and escape of macromolecules into microcirculation as occurs in extravasation, fluid shift and inflammation. They secrete chemical messengers such as nitric oxide (vasodilators) and endothelins (vasoconstrictors) and endothelial derived growth factors.

ARTERIES

- Arteries are vessels that conduct oxygen –rich blood (oxygenated blood) except pulmonary and umbilical arteries from the heart to the body tissues.
- Between the tunica adventitia and tunica media is elastic band rich in elastin.

Continuation
- Arteries have no valves except pulmonary artery and aorta.
- Arteries have thick walls and smaller luminal diameter than veins.
- They are the most flexible vessels. Increase in the diameter of arterial blood vessel is called vasodilation and decrease in diameter is called vasoconstriction.
- As the diameter of arteries increases, their tendency to oppose blood flow (**Peripheral vascular resistance**) decreases and vice versa.
- Old age and medical condition such as atherosclerosis bring about decrease in the elasticity of arteries.
- The lateral pressure exerted by contained column of blood on the arterial vessel is termed Arterial Blood Pressure.
- Arteries divide into smaller units called **arterioles.**

Continuation

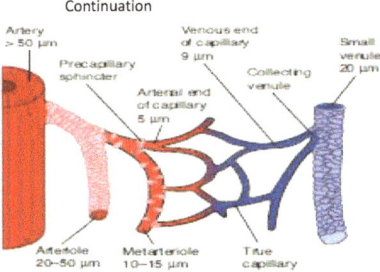

Figure 1:Blood vessels (Adapted from Review of Medical Physiology)

Continuation
- Arterioles are the site of resistance because they are narrower than arteries and they have more tunica media. Contraction of arterioles raises peripheral vascular resistance and reduces blood flow to the capillaries. They are therefore called **resistance blood vessel.**

VEINS
- Blood conduits to the heart.
- They have higher luminal diameter than arteries. Therefore they can hold more blood. They are called **capacitance blood vessel**. Phlebotomy is possible because of this reason and because of their superficial location.

Continuation
- Veins carry carbon dioxide rich blood except pulmonary and umbilical veins.
- Veins have valves. Contraction of muscles causes the proximal valve to open resulting in movement of blood into the heart. The rate at which venous blood reaches the right and left atria is called **venous return**. Occlusion of veins probably due to positive intrathoracic pressure as occurs during expiration reduces venous return and vice versa.
- Inflammation of veins is called phlebitis. Like arteries, air bubbles and clots can block the vascular lumen resulting in ischemia (reduction in tissue perfusion).
- Veins are made up of smaller units called **venules.**

CAPILLARIES
- The smallest blood vessels but with the greatest total cross sectional area.
- Depleted of tunica adventitia and tunica media.
- Forms an interface with the body cells.
- The diameter is 5µm at the arterial end and 9µm at the venous end (see Fig. 1).
- Formation and reabsorption of interstitial fluid depend on interplay of starling forces; the capillary hydrostatic pressure(CHP) and capillary oncotic pressure (COP). For interstitial fluid to be formed, CHP at arterial end >COP and for reabsorption, CHP at venous end<COP.

Continuation

- CHP at arterial end is 30mmHg, CHP at venous end is 15mmHg and COP is 25mmHg at both ends. Therefore, a pressure of 5mmHg favours formation while a pressure of 10mmHg favours reabsorption. Decreased in oncotic pressure due to liver diseases brings about increased risk of edema. COP at venous end increases in congestive heart failure and pulmonary heart disease resulting in increased chance of edema.
- Carbon dioxide rich blood is returned from parts above and below the heart by superior and inferior venacava.
- Oxygen rich blood leaves the heart through aorta. A force is required to drive blood to different regions of the body. This force is termed Arterial Blood Pressure.

(Figure has been removed due to copyright issues)

Figure 2: The human heart

HEART

- The heart is a muscular wedge shaped organ.
- Weighs about 300g and larger in adult male than adult female.
- Located in the middle midiastinum between T5 and T8 vertebral segments.
- It has 5 surfaces; anterior surface formed by right ventricle, posterior surface formed by left atrium, right pulmonary surface formed by right atrium, left pulmonary surface formed by left ventricle and diaphragmatic surface formed by right and left ventricles.

continuation

- It has 4 borders; superior border by right and left atria, inferior border by right and left ventricles, right border by right atrium and right ventricle and left border by left atrium and left ventricle.
- The heart is made up of three layers; the outer layer called the pericardium, the middle layer called the myocardium and the inner layer called the endocardium.
- The pericardium consists of the fibrous parietal and the inner visceral layer. In between these layers is a space filled with a serous fluid. The fluid reduces friction when the layers rub against each other as occurs during the cardiac cycle. The fluid is reabsorbed into the circulation. Accumulation of this fluid in this space occurs in pericarditis. Cardiac tamponade occurs when the accumulated fluid within the pericardium results in deranged tendency of the heart to stretch during diastole.

Continuation

- The myocardium consists of cardiac muscle and a specialized tissues that constitute the conduction system of the heart.
- The endocardium lines the cavity of the heart.
- The heart exhibits a mechanism through which it drives blood into the systemic circulation. This mechanism is known as the heartbeat. An average heart beat is 72/min. In a day, the heart beats 10,000times.
- The type of circulation in human beings is closed circulation.
- Circulations of blood between the heart and lungs and between the heart and aorta are known as pulmonary and systemic circulations respectively.

- The heart has blood flow controlling structures called valves. Examples are;

-Atrioventricular valves (tricuspid valve between right atrium and right ventricle auscultated at the left fifth intercostal space and bicuspid or mitral valve between left atrium and left ventricle auscultated at the left fifth intercostal space along mid-clavicular line).

- Semilunar valve (aortic valve between left ventricle and aorta auscultated at the right 2nd costal cartilage and pulmonary valve between right ventricle and pulmonary valve auscultated at the left 2nd costal cartilage). Semilunar valves are tricuspid.

BLOOD SUPPLY AND DRAINAGE

- The heart is supplied by coronary arteries.
- The right coronary artery (RCA) arises from anterior aortic sinus and left coronary artery (LCA) from left posterior aortic sinus.
- RCA supplies the right side of the heart and LCA, the left side.
- RCA branches into right marginal artery and posterior interventricular artery. The former supplies the superficial part of the right side of the heart and the latter branches into nodal artery that supplies conductive tissues (2/3 of the AV node). RCA also supplies the other parts of the right side of the heart including 1/3 of the interventricular septum.
- RCA unites (anastomosis) with the circumflex artery at the coronary sulcus.

Continuation
- The anastomosis of the heart is anatomical not a functional type and therefore, narrowing of the arterial vessels supplying the heart could result in myocardial infarction.
- LCA supplies the left side of the heart.
- LCA gives rise to anterior interventricular artery and circumflex artery.
- Anterior interventricular artery supplies the remaining 2/3 of the interventricular septum.
- Circumflex artery branches into nodal artery that supplies the remaining 1/3 of AV node.
- Circumflex artery branches into left marginal artery which supplies the superficial part of the left side of the heart.

Continuation
- Anterior interventricular artery unites with posterior interventricular artery at the interventricular groove.
- The right and left septal branches also unite at interventricular septum.
- The myocardium receives arterial supply during diastole.
- The proportion of the cardiac output received by the heart is 4.8%.
- Venous drainage is through small, middle and great cardiac veins. These veins drain into the right atrium through coronary sinus.
- Lymphatic drainage is by tracheobronchial lymph node.

NERVOUS SUPPLY

- The heart is innervated by sympathetic (adrenergic) fibers and parasympathetic (vagal) fibers.
- Adrenergic nerve fiber to the heart is epicardial. Stimulation of β1 and β2 adrenergic receptors results in cyclic adenosine monophosphate (CAMP)- mediated increase in force of contraction (positive inotropic action) and increase in heart rate (positive chronotropic action).
- Vagal fibers are subendocardial. Stimulation of muscarinic cholinergic receptor (M2 receptors) causes CAMP-mediated decrease in heart rate
- Reciprocal innervation occurs in the heart.

(Figure has been removed due to copyright issues)

Figure 3: electrical events of the cardiac muscle (Adapted from Review of Medical Physiology)

(Figure has been removed due to copyright issues)

Figure 4: electrical events of the pacemaker tissue (Adapted from Review of Medical Physiology)

PACEMAKER AND CARDIAC MUSCLE POTENTIALS

- Influx of sodium ions contributes to the first phase of pacemaker potential and such channels are called H channels.
- Influx of calcium ions through slow opening calcium channel is responsible for the pacemaker action potential.

- As far as cardiac muscle is concerned, depolarization is due to influx of sodium ions through the fast opening sodium channels.
- Initial repolarization is due to inactivation of sodium channels.
- Plateau is due to influx of slow opening calcium channels.
- Hyperpolarization is due to net efflux of potassium channels.

CONDUCTION SYSTEM OF THE HEART

- Denervation of the heart does not make the heart to stop beating. This is due to the presence of specialized tissue called sinoatrial node (SA node), the primary pacemaker tissue located in the right atrium at the opening of superior venacava which is capable of generating electrical impulses spontaneously at a higher rate.
- Impulses from SA node spreads to the AV node (located in posterior interatrial septum) through purkinje typed internodal tract (which include the anterior fibers of bachman, middle fibers of wenchebach and posterior fibers of thorel).

(Figure has been removed due to copyright issues)

Figure 5: Cardiac conduction system (Adapted from Review of Medical Physiology)

continuation
- In the AV node, conduction is slow (0.05m/s). This known as AV nodal delay allows atrial contraction to precede ventricular contraction. It also allows ventricular filling to precede ventricular ejection.
- Impulses from AV bode reach the left and right ventricle through left bundle of His and right bundle of His.
- The bundle of His and the branches transmit impulses to rapidly conducting purkinje fibers (4m/s) which run subendocardially and end on myocardial cells.

Continuation
- Depolarization begins at the left side of interventricular septum and spreads towards the right side.
- Impulses converge on the apex of the heart (located in the left V intercostal space along the mid-clavicular line).
- Pulmonary conus and the posterior basal portion of the interventricular septum are the last parts to be depolarized

ELECTROCARDIOGRAM

- The recording of the electrical activities of the heart taken from the surface of the body is called electrocardiogram.
- Invented by Willem Einthoven.
- There are three bipolar (standard) limb leads and nine unipolar leads (3 augumented limb leads and 6 precordial leads or chest leads).

(Figure has been removed due to copyright issues.)

Figure 5: electrocardiograph

- Converts electrical impulses to understandable language (ECG waves).
- The amplitude and duration of ECG waves have a wide clinical implication.
- P wave (0.1s, 0.1mV) is due to atrial depolarization.
- QRS (0.08s)complex is due to ventricular depolarization.
- T (0.32s) wave is due to ventricular repolarization.
- ECG intervals includes PR (0.18-0.2s) interval, measures the spread of electrical activities from atria to ventricles.

- QT interval (0.42s) measures the spread of electrical activities through ventricle.
- R-R interval is d interval btw the peak of two adjacent ECG waves. Exercise, emotion shortens it.
- Heart rate=300/no of large boxes between R-R interval or 10 x ECG cycles in a 6 s strip.
- ST interval is isoelectric. Elevation occurs in myocardial infarction and depression is seen in myocardial ischemia.

(Figures have been removed due to copyright issues.)

Figure 6: electrocardiogram

Figure 7: electrocardiogram

Figure 8: electrocardiogram

Figure 9: ECG recorded from the six chest leads

Figure 10; ECG recorded from the three augumented limb leads

APPLICATIONS
ECG changes with change in heart rate

SINUS TACHYCARDIA (LEAD I) short R-R interval

(Figure has been removed due to copyright issues.)

Figure 11; sinus bradycardia (LEAD III) short R-R interval

HEART BLOCK (PROLONGED PR INTERVAL)

MYOCARDIA ISCHEMIA (DEPRESSED ST SEGMENT)

(Figure has been removed due to copyright issues.)

Figure 12; Applications of ECG

MECHANICAL EVENTS OF THE HEART

- Cardiac cycle is a coordinated sequence of mechanical events during each heart beat.
- It is 0.8 seconds at normal heart beat and decreased by sympathetic stimulation.
- Consists of diastole (.53s) and systole (.27).
- Diastole consists of protodiastole, atrial systole, isometric relaxation and filling phases.

ECG waves	Implications
Atrial depolarization (P waves)	Atrial contraction (atrial systole)
Ventricular depolarization (QRS) (systole)	Ventricular contraction
Ventricular repolarization (T waves)	Ventricular relaxation

•Atrial repolarization merges with QRS complex on an ECG strip.

•Atrial repolarization produces atrial relaxation or atrial diastole.

Systole consists of isometric contraction and ejection period.

CARDIAC OUTPUT

•Cardiac output is the volume of blood ejected by each ventricle per minute. It is about 5L/min.

Continuation.

- According to Frank-Starling law, Cardiac output=**Stroke volume** x **Heart rate**
- Heart rate is the number of beats produced by the heart per minute.
- It represents the number of times left ventricle contracts to eject blood per mInute.
- Originates from the sinoatrial node.
- It is about 72 beats/minutes in adult man at rest and this is called *sinus rhythm.*
- Increased and depressed by sympathetic and vagal stimulation respectively.
- Actions relating to heart rate and force of contraction are called chronotropic and inotropic actions respectively.

- Heart rate (HR) is controlled in the medulla by dorsal motor nucleus and nucleus ambiguus.
- Decrease and increase in heart rate originating from SA node are called sinus bradycardia and sinus tachycardia.
- Sleep may lead to sinus bradycardia.
- Pregnancy, exercise and anxiety may lead to sinus tachycardia.
- Pulsation is the use of sense of touch to judge the heart rate in peripheral arteries. Or the palpation of heart rate in arteries that are constricted by bone using a well trained fingertips.
- Pulse rate is the number of times arteries oscillate per minute.
- HR may be more than pulse rate. This is known as pulsus deficit.

PULSATION SITES

Pulse can be felt in
- Superficial temporal artery
- Facial artery
- Right and left common carotid arteries
- Apex of the heart
- Brachial artery
- Radial artery
- Femoral artery
- Popliteal artery
- Dorsal pedalis artery
- Posterior tibial artery
- Fontanels in neonates

FACTORS AFFECTING PULSE RATE

- Age; Pulse rate is higher in neonate than old people.
- Sex; Pubertal males have higher pulse rate than female.
- State of activity; exercise increases pulse rate, sleep decreases pulse rate.
- Anxiety increases pulse rate.
- In pregnancy, there is increase in pulse rate.
- Circadian variation; it is higher in day than night.
- Temperature: high temperature increases pulse rate.

Continuation
- End diastolic volume or preload is the amount of blood in each ventricle at the end of diastole. It is 130ml. In restrictive cardiomyopathy, it may be greatly reduced.
- Stroke volume is the volume of blood ejected by each ventricle per beat.
- It is 70ml/beat.
- Stroke volume is affected by contractility, End diastolic volume, peripheral resistance, etc.
- Stroke volume/End diastolic volume =Ejection fraction. i.e 70/130x100%
- Ejection fraction is 45-60%. In congestive cardiomyopathy, the fraction may be lower than 40%.

FACTORS AFFECTING CARDIAC OUTPUT (CO)

- Posture; sudden standing decreases CO. In untrained people, prolonged standing exacerbates the decrease. Suppination and pronation have no effect.
- Muscular exercise increases co
- Hemorrhage most especially heavy hemorrhage and chronic light hemorrhage decreases co
- Obesity and large body surface area increase co
- Negative intrathoracic pressure (eg inspiration) increases co and positive intrathoracic pressure decreases it
- Anatomical anomaly like kyphosis may decrease co.
- Dietary factor (as in high salt) intake increases co
- Emotion such as anxiety increases co

HEART SOUNDS

- Noises (vibrations) produced by heartbeat, valvular closure, flow of blood and arterial elastic recoil.
- The noises reflect turbulence flow of blood.
- Heart sounds can be measured by stethoscope and other devices.

HEART SOUNDS (cont'd)

- There are four heart sounds.
- The first heart sound S1 is due majorly to the vibration set up by the simultaneous closure of the atrioventricular valves.
- It is long, soft and low pitched resembling the word "LUB".

HEART SOUNDS (cont'd)

- It is 25-40HZ in frequency and 10-17s . It has mitral and tricuspid components.
- Second heart sound S2 is high pitched and short resembling the word 'DUB'.
- Has aortic and pulmonary components.
- Second heart sound S2 is due to vibrations set up by the sudden closure of semilunar valves.

I

HEART SOUNDS (cont'd)
- S1 and S2 can be measured using stethoscope.
- S3 and S4 are extra heartbeat. They are low pitched.
- S3 is soft.
- Occurrence of S3 is pathological in people above 40 years.
- Occurrence of S4 is pathological.
- S4 is also low pitched and soft.

ABNORMAL HEART SOUNDS
- Murmurs are abnormal noises generated within the cardiovascular system.
- Abnormal noises produced outside the cardiovascular system are called bruits.
- Murmurs may be due to valvular incompetence (weak valves leading to regurgitation of blood) and stenosis (narrowing).

ABNORMAL HEART SOUNDS (cont'd)

- Diastolic murmurs are due to incompetence of semilunar valve, stenosis of atrioventricular valve, and anemia.
- Systolic murmurs are due to incompetence of the atrioventricular valve and stenosis of semilunar valve.
- Continuous murmurs are due to patent ductus arteriosus.

BLOOD PRESSURE (BP) AND ITS REGULATION

- The lateral pressure exerted by a contained column of blood on the heart.
- Measured non-invasively via sphygmomanometer using procedure that was invented by Nicolai Korotkoff.
- BP is expressed as systolic blood pressure (SBP)/diastolic blood pressure (DBP).
- The difference between SBP and DBP is called pulse pressure.

Cont of blood pressure and its regulation
- The average arterial blood pressure is called mean arterial blood pressure (MAP).
- MAP = DBP +1/3(Pulse pressure).
- Any factor that raises DBP has a great influence on MAP.
- Peripheral resistance (PR) is the opposition to the flow of blood
- PR is inversely proportional to vascular radius
- MAP =cardiac output x PR.
- In atherosclerosis, PR increases resulting in increase in MAP.
- Chronic salt loading as in habitual consumption of high salt diet increases blood volume and cardiac output leading to a rise in MAP

- In adult, the normal blood pressure is 90-120/60-80.
- Sustained increase and decrease in BP are called hypertension and hypotension.
- Variation in BP could be due to;
-Circadian variation; BP is higher in afternoon than morning.
-Age; old people have higher blood pressure than the children

FACTORS AFFECTING BLOOD PRESSURE
-Sex; Pubertal males due to androgens have higher BP than female
- Moderate rise in temperature increases BP
- Emotion such as anxiety increase BP

(cont. of factors affecting blood pressure)
- BP increases after meal.
- Menstruation increases BP.
- Posture, eg sudden standing decreases BP (postural or orthostatic hypotension). Suppination and pronation may not affect blood pressure.
- In pregnancy, BP decreases due to diversion of blood to the reproductive structures.
- High salt intake raises BP.
- Lifestyle such as alcoholism ,smoking and sedation raises BP.
- Muscular activities increases systolic pressure and reduces diastolic pressure such that the mean arterial pressure does not change .

REGULATION OF BLOOD PRESSURE

- Blood pressure is controlled on a short term basis by **baroreceptors and kidney renin angiotensin aldosterone system** on long term basis.
- Baroreceptors are uncapsulated nerve endings located in carotid sinus, aortic arch, right atrium, left ventricles and the lungs.
- Their stimulations reflexly decrease blood pressure.

BLOOD PRESSURE AND ITS REGULATION

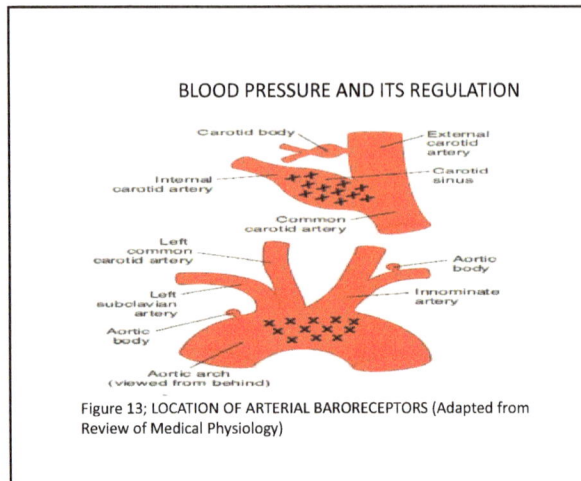

Figure 13; LOCATION OF ARTERIAL BARORECEPTORS (Adapted from Review of Medical Physiology)

BLOOD PRESSURE AND ITS REGULATION

Baroreceptors are controlled in the medulla (brainstem)

Figure 14; BP control (Adapted from Review of Medical Physiology)

24

BLOOD PRESSURE AND ITS REGULATION

RENIN ANGIOTENSIN ALDOSTERONE SYSTEM

- The most powerful blood pressure regulatory mechanism.
- A compensatory mechanism to acute hemorrhage .
- Low blood pressure->Renin->angiotensin I ->angiotensin II->Aldosterone->Na and water retention->ECF expansion->high blood pressure->Atrial Natriuretic

  Peptide-> Na and water excretion -> normal BP

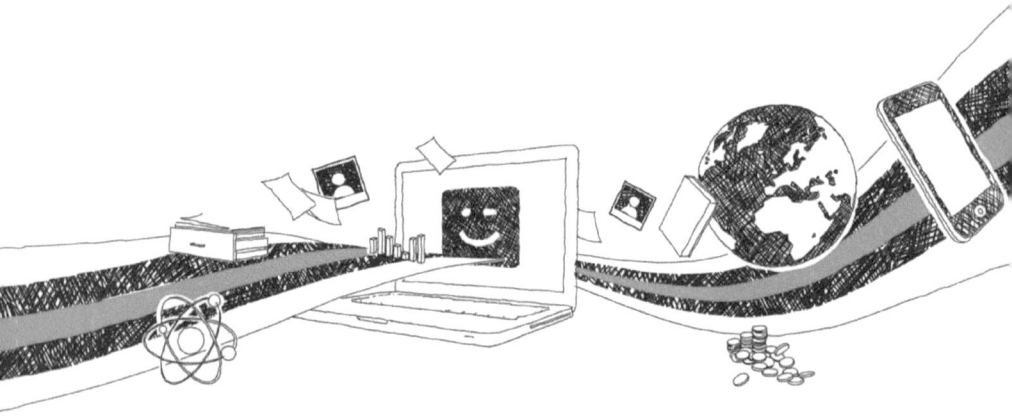
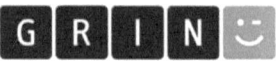